The Kids' Guide to
Disease & Wellness
Why People Get Sick & How They Can Stay Well

AIDS & HIV

The Facts for Kids

Rae Simons

The Kids' Guide to Disease & Wellness:
Why People Get Sick and How They Can Stay Well
AIDS & HIV: The Facts for Kids

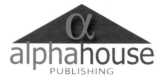

AlphaHouse Publishing
201 Harding Avenue
Vestal, NY 13850

First Printing

9 8 7 6 5 4 3 2 1

ISBN: 978-1-934970-20-1
ISBN (series): 978-1-934970-11-9
    Library of Congress Control Number: 2008930679

Author: Simons, Rae

Cover design by MK Bassett-Harvey.
Interior design by MK Bassett-Harvey and Wendy Arakawa.

Printed in India by International Print-O-Pac Limited

An ISO 9001 Company

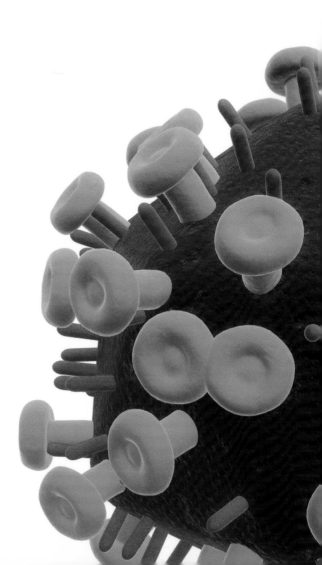

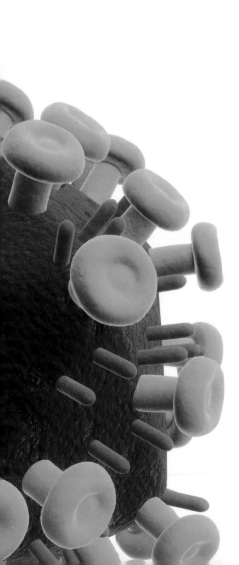

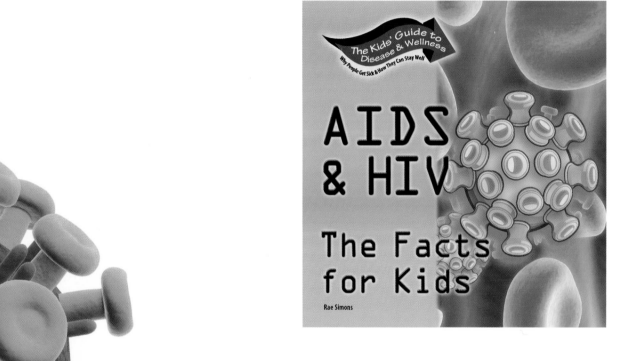

The Kids' Guide to
Disease & Wellness
Why People Get Sick & How They Can Stay Well

AIDS & HIV

The Facts for Kids

Rae Simons

By Rae Simons

Series List

Introduction

According to a recent study reported in the Virginia Henderson International Nursing Library, kids worry about getting sick. They worry about AIDS and cancer, about allergies and the "super-germs" that resist medication. They know about these ills—but they don't always understand what causes them or how they can be prevented.

Unfortunately, most 9- to 11–year–olds, the study found, get their information about diseases like AIDS from friends and television; only 20 percent of the children interviewed based their understanding of illness on facts they had learned at school. Too often, kids believe urban legends, schoolyard folktales, and exaggerated movie plots. Oftentimes, misinformation like this only makes their worries worse. The January 2008 *Child Health News* reported that 55 percent of all children between 9 and 13 "worry almost all the time" about illness.

This series, **The Kids' Guide to Disease and Wellness**, offers readers clear information on various illnesses and conditions, as well as the immunizations that can prevent many diseases. The books dispel the myths with clearly presented facts and colorful, accurate illustrations. Better yet, these books will help kids understand not only illness—but also what they can do to stay as healthy as possible.

—*Dr. Elise Berlan*

Just The Facts

- AIDS (Acquired Immunodeficiency Syndrome) is a disease that is caused by HIV(Human Immunodeficiency Virus)

- HIV hurts your immune system so it can't fight off diseases, including diseases that wouldn't otherwise hurt you.

- You can get AIDS from infected body fluids. You can be exposed to these a lot of different ways, including by using a needle that was used by someone with AIDS, or having unprotected sex with an infected person. AIDS can also be passed from mother to child.

- You cannot get AIDS by giving blood, being touched by or breathed on by an infected person, or touching things an infected person touched, as long as you don't touch their body fluids.

- HIV can often be in a person's body for years before it is noticed.

- The only way to be sure you have AIDS is to be tested by a doctor.

- Scientific research has made it possible to live for years with AIDS. However, scientists continue to look for new treatments, as well as a vaccine for the disease.

- Although AIDS is a problem around the world, it is worst in Africa and Asia, where many people live in poverty and cannot afford treatment for the disease.

What Is AIDS?

You hear a lot about AIDS and HIV these days. You may have seen television shows and movies where characters had this disease. You might hear about it at school. You may even know someone who has it. You may think it's connected somehow to homosexuals. But lots of kids—and adults, too—don't really understand what HIV/AIDS is. They don't know how you catch it, who gets it, or what causes it. Lots of people don't even know what these letters stand for: **A**cquired **I**mmuno**D**eficiency **S**yndrome—AIDS—got its name because:

It is acquired; in other words, it's something that has to be passed to you from another person. It is not handed down genetically; it cannot be passed down to you from your parents. This means if your boyfriend has AIDS you could catch it from him—but if your grandmother who lives in another country has AIDS, you're not going to discover that she passed it on to you.

8

It affects the body's **immune** system, the part of the body that fights off diseases.

It is considered a **deficiency** because it makes the immune system stop working the way it should.

At first doctors thought it was a **syndrome** (and not a disease) because people with AIDS have a number of different symptoms and diseases.

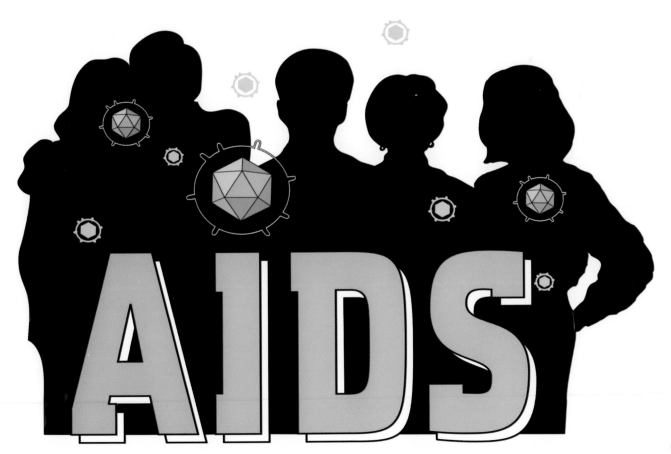

What Is HIV?

Today, doctors think that "HIV disease" is a better name. HIV stands for Human Immunodeficiency Virus. It's the virus that causes AIDS. People can have the HIV virus (shown here) inside their bodies, but not seem sick.

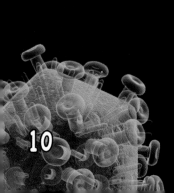

10

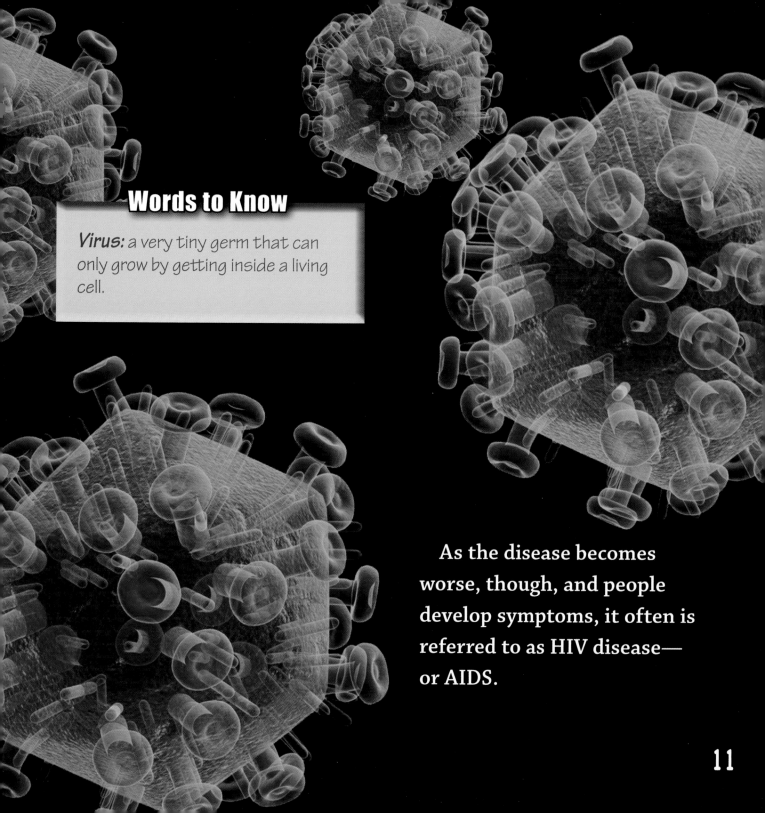

As the disease becomes worse, though, and people develop symptoms, it often is referred to as HIV disease— or AIDS.

Where Did HIV/AIDS Come From?

Scientists believe that HIV began in chimpanzees in Africa. The virus was probably spread to humans when the chimpanzees were killed for their meat. Blood from the animals got into the hunters' wounds—and the first people caught the virus.

Scientists and doctors gave HIV/AIDS its name in the 1980s when the first people started getting sick with it. At the beginning, many patients were homosexual men —which made some people think this was a "homosexual problem."

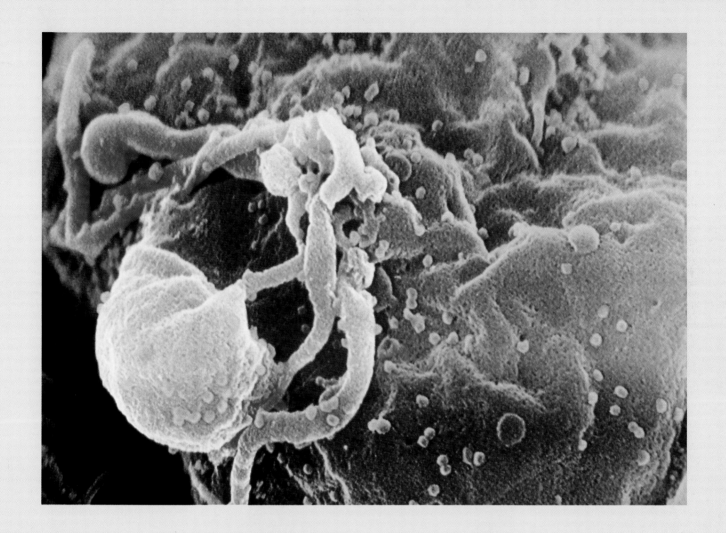

Words to Know

Homosexual: a person who is attracted sexually to a member of the same sex. Male homosexuals are attracted to males, female homosexuals to females.

Before long, doctors realized other people were getting sick with HIV and AIDS, too. Doctors know now that AIDS is an "everybody" problem.

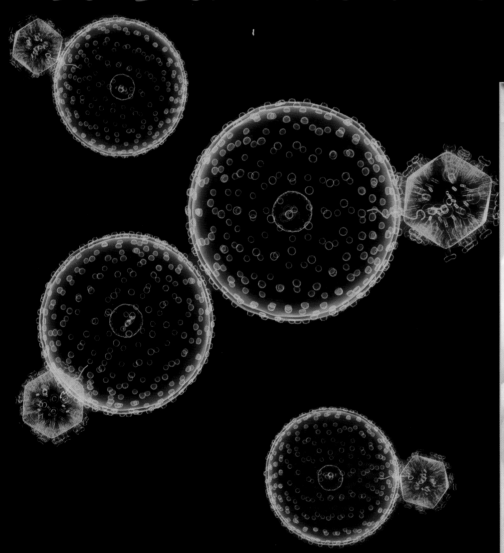

What Does HIV/AIDS Do Inside Your Body?

ASK THE DOCTOR

My brother says he's afraid he has AIDS. But wouldn't he feel sick if he had AIDS?

A: A few people will have AIDS within a few months from the time they are first exposed to HIV, but that's not usual. In most people, symptoms do not show up for ten to twelve years. If your brother thinks he may have been exposed to HIV, it's very important that he see a doctor right away. If he does have HIV, the sooner he knows, the sooner he can begin treatment.

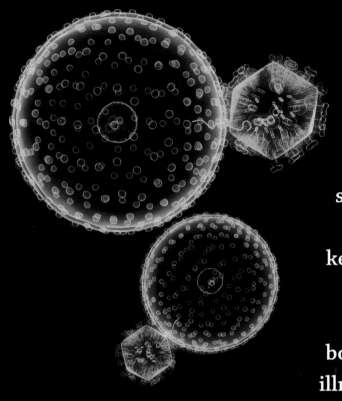

The worst thing about AIDS is that it hurts your immune system—the special cells in your blood that fight off germs and keep you from getting sick. When this happens, you can get sick with other infections, and your body won't be able to fight off the illness. People with AIDS often die from another disease (such as pneumonia or cancer).

Words to Know

Pneumonia: an infection in the lungs.

All the places where HIV can make you sick on the OUTSIDE:

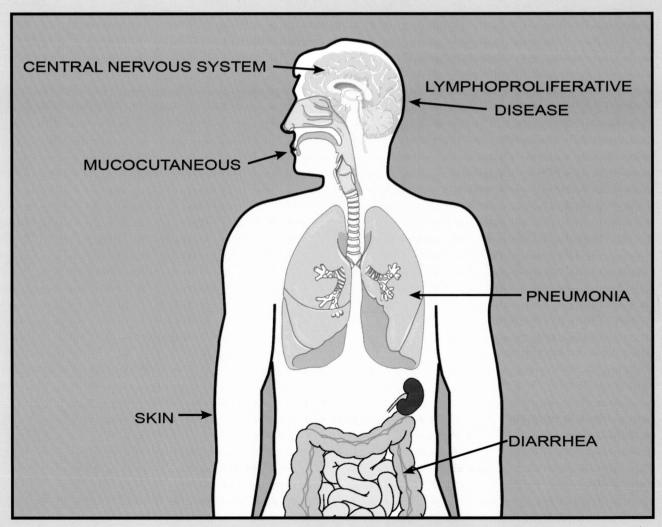

When a virus or bacteria (what we often call germs) gets into your body through a cut, through the air you breathe, or through something you've eaten, special cells in your blood, white blood cells called helper T cells, get busy. They pass along the message to another group of white blood cells—B cells—telling them to make the weapons (called antibodies) they need to kill the germs. If a virus or bacteria makes its way past the antibodies, it can cause an infection. When that happens, a different type of T cell recognizes the change in the infected cell and kills it. This prevents the infection from spreading. At least this is what is *supposed* to happen. But when someone has HIV, eventually she will no longer be able to fight off infections that other people have no problem resisting.

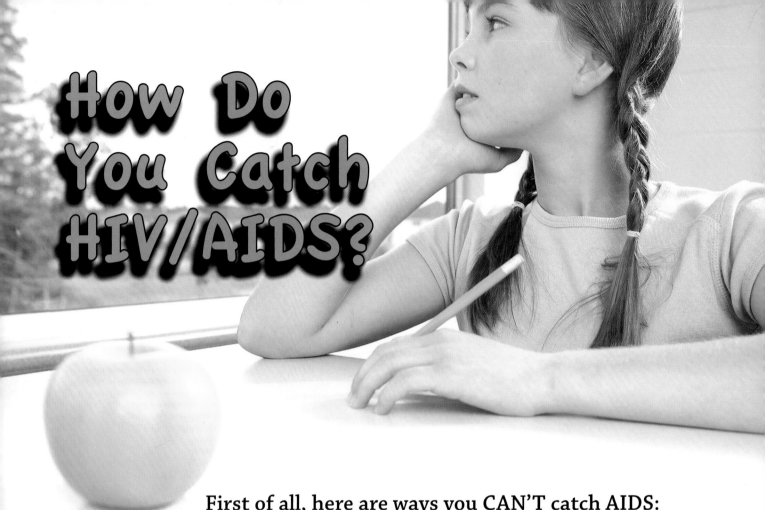

How Do You Catch HIV/AIDS?

First of all, here are ways you CAN'T catch AIDS:

You can't catch AIDS from being in the same room with someone who has HIV/AIDS.

You can't catch AIDS from touching something that someone with HIV/AIDS has touched.

You can't catch AIDS from breathing the same air as someone with HIV/AIDS.

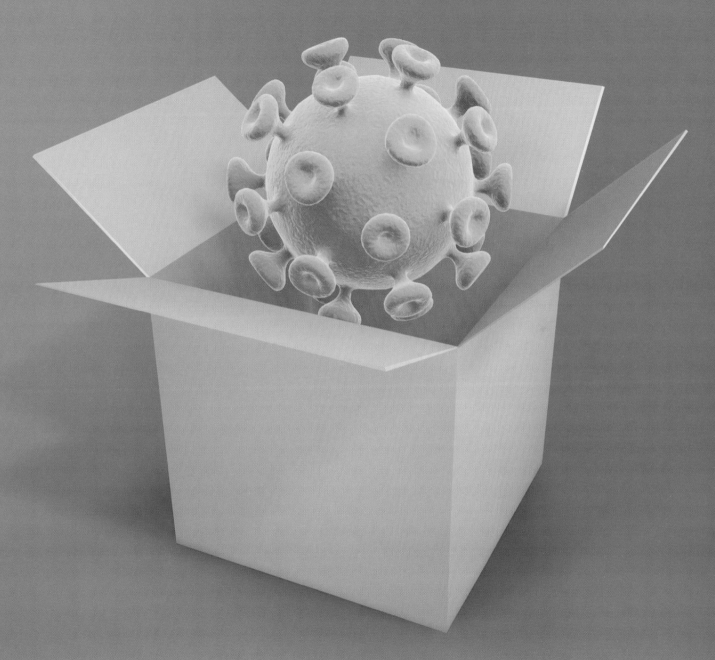

The ONLY way to catch HIV/AIDS is through certain body fluids.

Sex

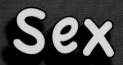

The most common way to catch HIV is through unprotected sexual intercourse. This means any kind of sex, not just sex between two homosexuals.

Words to Know

Unprotected sex: when people have sex with each other without using a condom. A condom is like a tight rubber glove that fits over the man's penis and keeps his semen—the fluid that comes out of his penis when he has sex—from escaping.

21

Blood

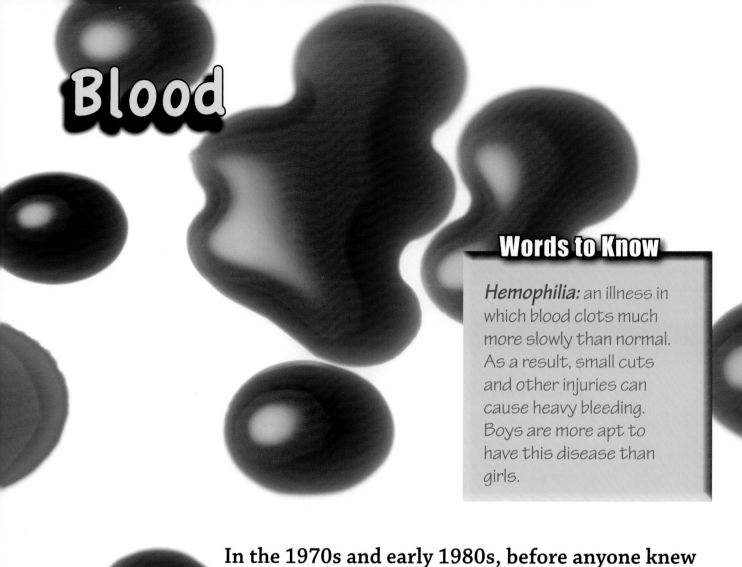

In the 1970s and early 1980s, before anyone knew very much about HIV/AIDS, blood donors who didn't know they had the disease gave their blood to hospitals and at Red Cross blood drives—and the virus got into the blood supply that was given out to sick or injured people who needed blood.

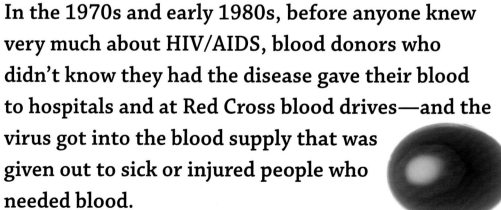

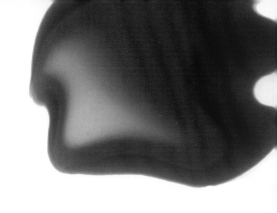

Eventually, doctors realized that some people were catching HIV/AIDS from blood transfusions. Beginning in 1985, the blood supply has been tested for HIV, and there is no longer much risk that someone will get HIV/AIDS from a blood transfusion. However, people who received transfusions between 1975 and 1985 had a high risk of getting the infected blood. Among the people most at risk are those with hemophilia. People with hemophilia use blood to control bleeding episodes. Between 1975 and 1985, as many as half of the people with hemophilia were infected with HIV through blood.

Dirty Drug Needles

Some drug users inject the drug into their veins with a hypodermic needle like the one shown here. Hypodermic needles cost money, and drug users often spend most of their money on drugs. They don't want to spend money on needles, so they often share them.

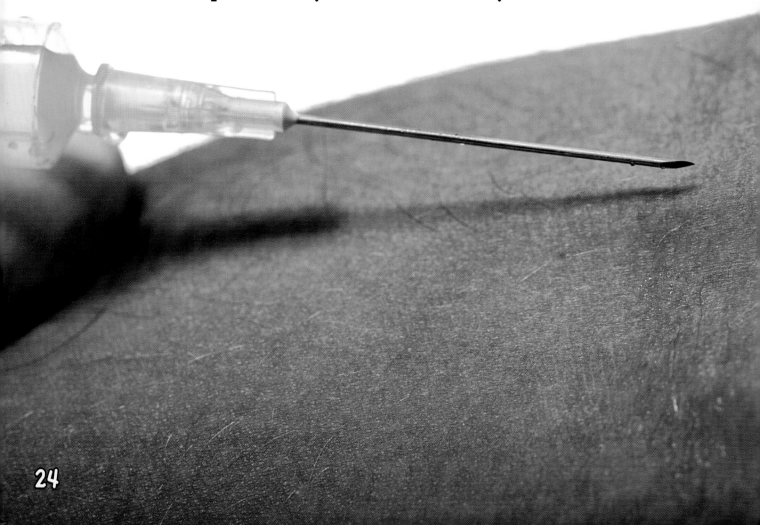

When drug users share needles, some blood from the last user often stays on the used needle. If that person had HIV in his blood, the next person to use the needle will be injecting the virus along with the drug into his blood. This makes intravenous drug users another group of people who are at high risk of catching HIV/AIDS.

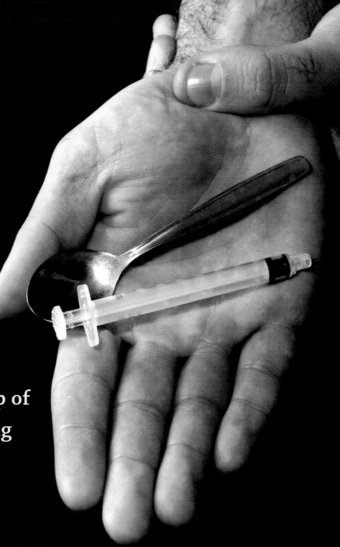

Words to Know

Inject: to force or push a fluid into something else.

Mother to Child

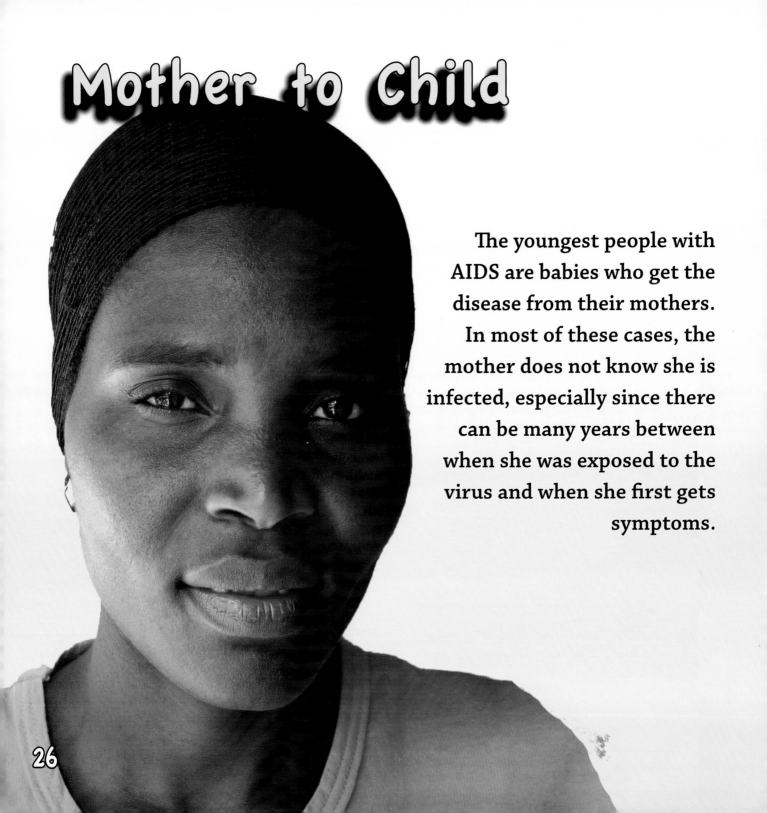

The youngest people with AIDS are babies who get the disease from their mothers. In most of these cases, the mother does not know she is infected, especially since there can be many years between when she was exposed to the virus and when she first gets symptoms.

If there is any chance a woman has been exposed to HIV, she should be tested for the virus before becoming pregnant. Medicine can be given to pregnant women with HIV to protect their babies during pregnancy. After the baby is born, women with HIV should not breastfeed, so that the virus isn't passed to their babies through breast milk.

Words to Know

Exposed: put in a position where there is no protection or shield against a danger or disease.

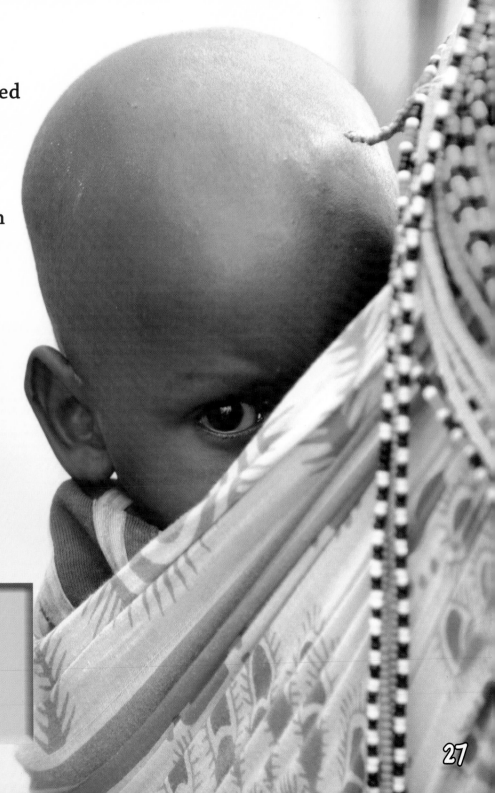

27

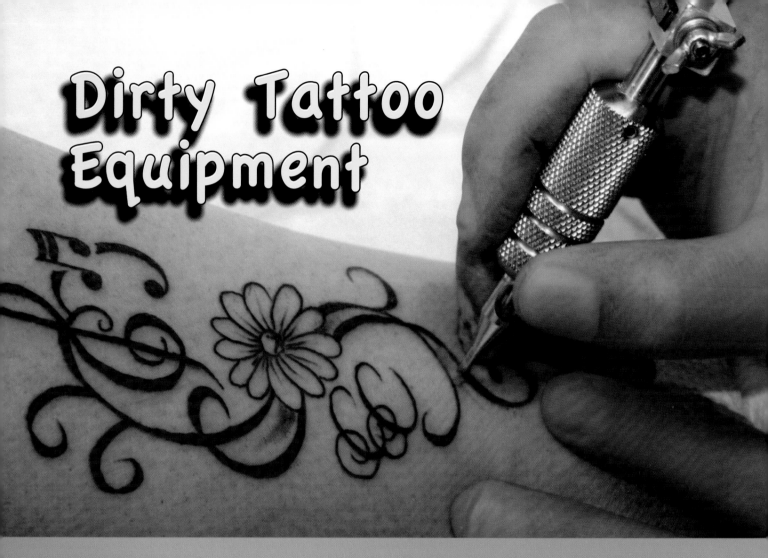

Dirty Tattoo Equipment

Tattoos are becoming more and more popular, especially among young people. But the needles used for tattooing (and also for body piercing) can carry HIV. In that case, when the needle pierces your skin to inject the dye, it may also be injecting HIV into your blood.

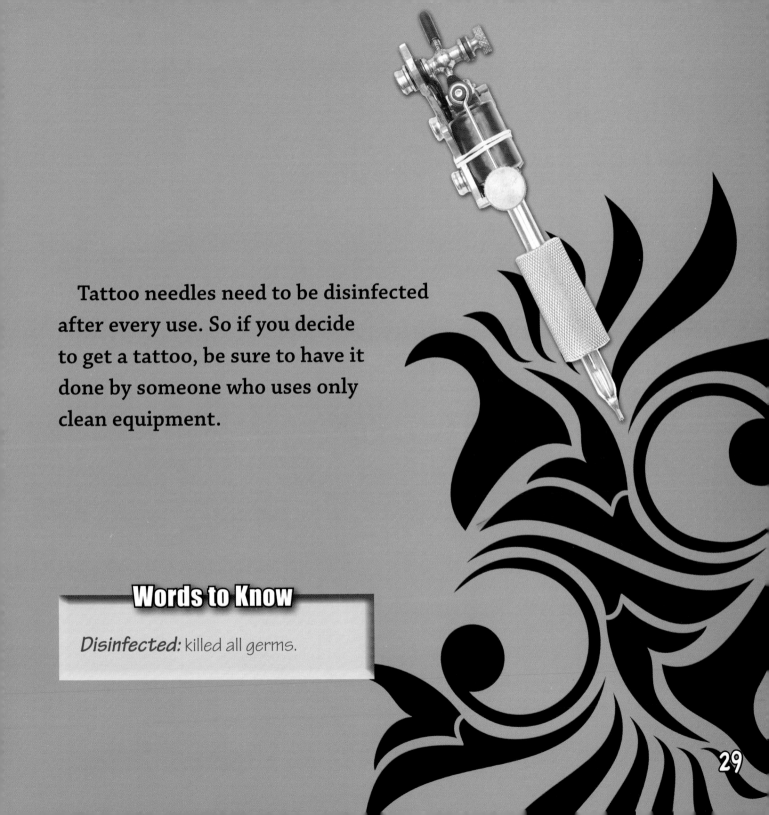

Tattoo needles need to be disinfected after every use. So if you decide to get a tattoo, be sure to have it done by someone who uses only clean equipment.

Words to Know

Disinfected: killed all germs.

How Do You Know If You Have HIV/AIDS?

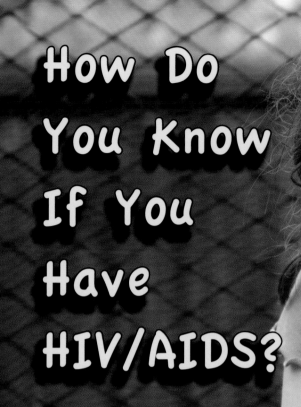

The only way to know for sure if you have HIV is to go to the doctor and get a blood test. The blood test will check to see if you have the antibodies in your blood that your body creates to fight the virus. If you do have these antibodies, it means that HIV is present in your blood. This means you have HIV.

ASK THE DOCTOR

My sister's friend got tested for HIV and it came back negative—but the doctor says she has to go back for another test in a few months. How come?

A: It takes a while for your body to create enough HIV antibodies to show up on the blood test. To be safe, doctors often ask people to come back for a second or even a third test, especially if there's a good chance the person was exposed to HIV. It's better to be absolutely certain.

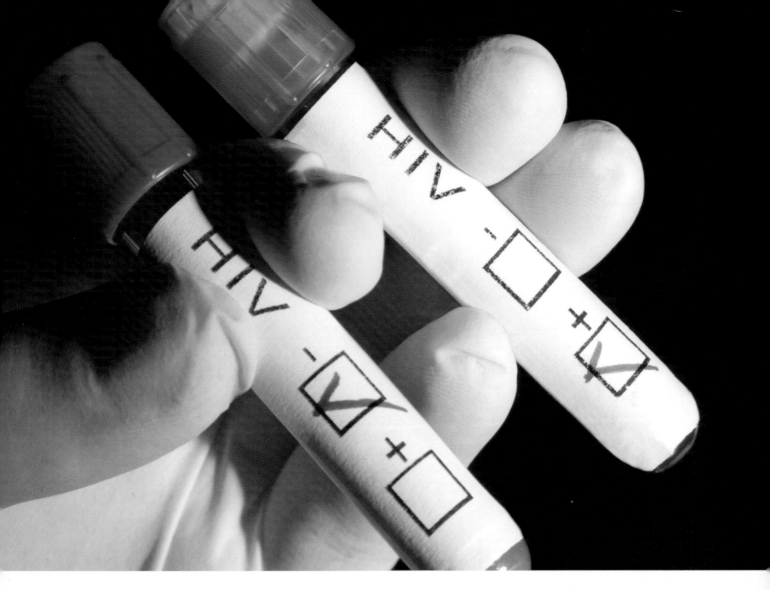

Just because you have HIV, though, doesn't mean you have AIDS. Doctors only say a person has AIDS once he has tested positive for HIV in his blood, he has had one or more AIDS-related infections or illnesses, and the number of helper T cells in his blood has reached or fallen below a certain level.

What Happens If You Have HIV?

Up until recently, if you found out you had HIV, you knew you would die soon. Today, however, some people who have the virus have still not developed AIDS even after many years. AIDS has no cure yet, but many people with HIV are living longer and staying healthier. New medicines have made this possible.

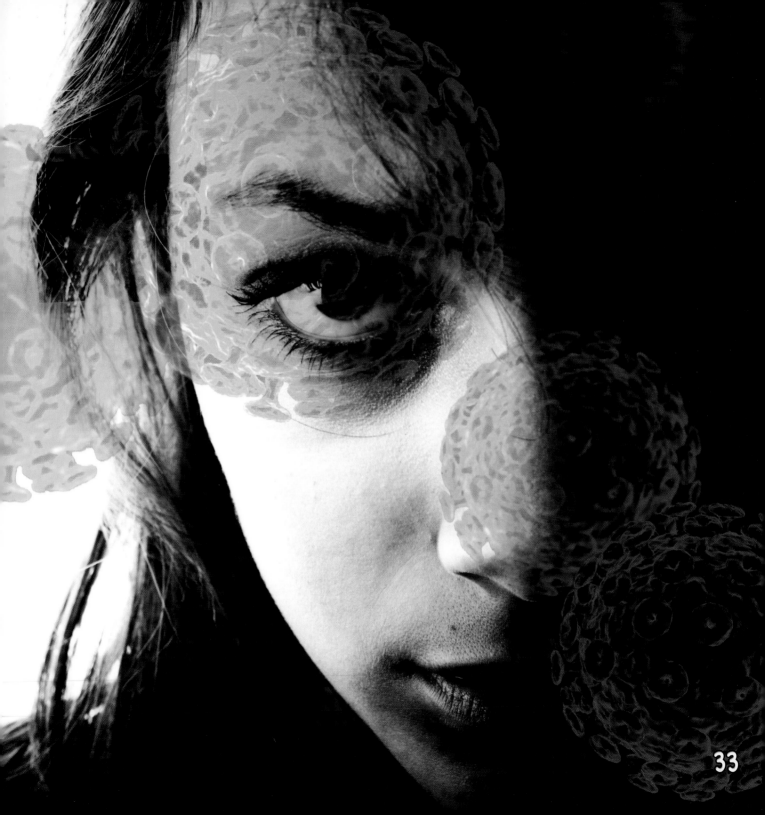

Treatment for HIV/AIDS

Scientists have not found a cure for AIDS yet, but they have found new and powerful drugs that allow people to stay healthy longer. For many people living with HIV/AIDS, a single medicine does not work. Most take a combination of many drugs. They work together to reduce the level of HIV in the body, allowing the body's own T-helper cells to return to healthier levels.

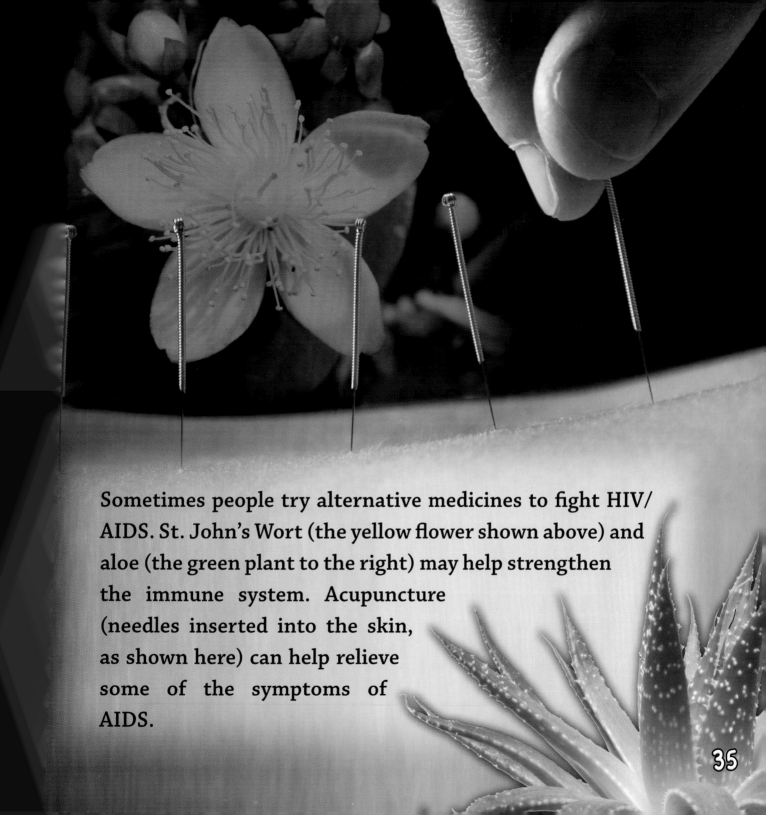

Sometimes people try alternative medicines to fight HIV/AIDS. St. John's Wort (the yellow flower shown above) and aloe (the green plant to the right) may help strengthen the immune system. Acupuncture (needles inserted into the skin, as shown here) can help relieve some of the symptoms of AIDS.

What Is HIV/AIDS Doing to the World?

The worst problem with the medicines used to treat AIDS is that they are very expensive. Around the world, many of the people living with HIV/AIDS are also living in poverty. They may have no money to buy the medicine or even go to the doctor. They may live in a region so poor that they don't even have a doctor or clinic nearby where they could go if they did have money.

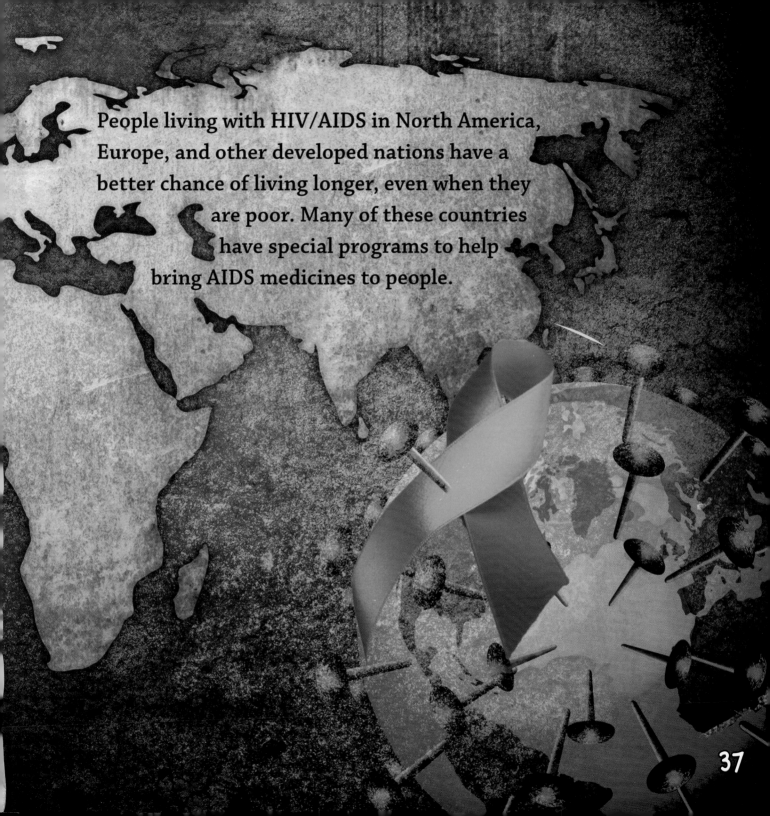

People living with HIV/AIDS in North America, Europe, and other developed nations have a better chance of living longer, even when they are poor. Many of these countries have special programs to help bring AIDS medicines to people.

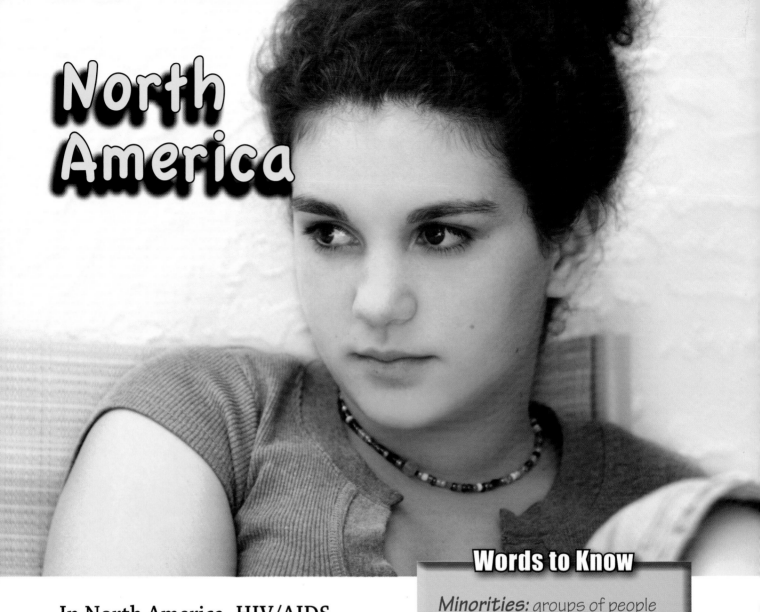

North America

In North America, HIV/AIDS is worse for blacks and other minorities than it is for whites.

Words to Know

Minorities: groups of people who are different from the larger group to which they belong.

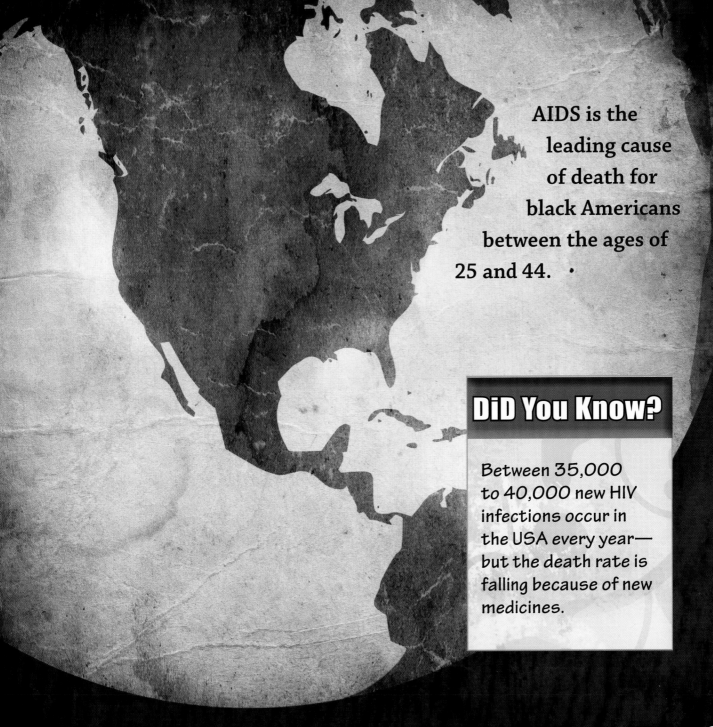

AIDS is the leading cause of death for black Americans between the ages of 25 and 44.

DiD You Know?

Between 35,000 to 40,000 new HIV infections occur in the USA every year—but the death rate is falling because of new medicines.

Africa

In Africa, HIV has touched the lives of more than a quarter of the population. This means that one of every four people either has HIV/AIDS or has a household member with the disease. Almost everyone has a neighbor, a teacher, a friend, or a relative who is sick or dying.

DiD You Know?

Africa is home to just over 10% of the world's population but more than 60% of all the people in the world living with HIV live there.

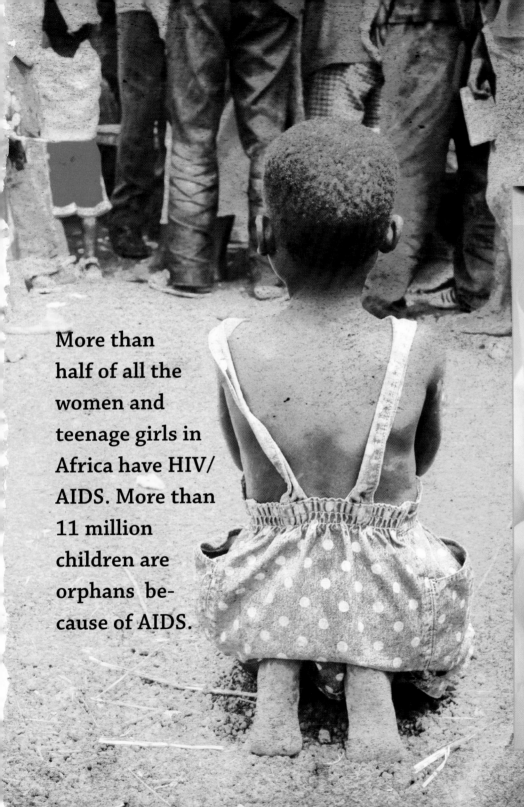

More than half of all the women and teenage girls in Africa have HIV/AIDS. More than 11 million children are orphans be-cause of AIDS.

ASK THE DOCTOR

Do people in Africa get a different kind of AIDS than people in the rest of the world?

A: No, AIDS is always caused by HIV, and the ways HIV passes from person to person are exactly the same in all parts of the world. There may be some different strains of HIV in Africa, but the virus is basically the same as it is in the rest of the world. What's different about Africa is how poor it is, and how many other diseases there are. This means that people with AIDS are less likely to get anti-retroviral medicine and antibiotics and may be exposed to many germs they cannot resist.

41

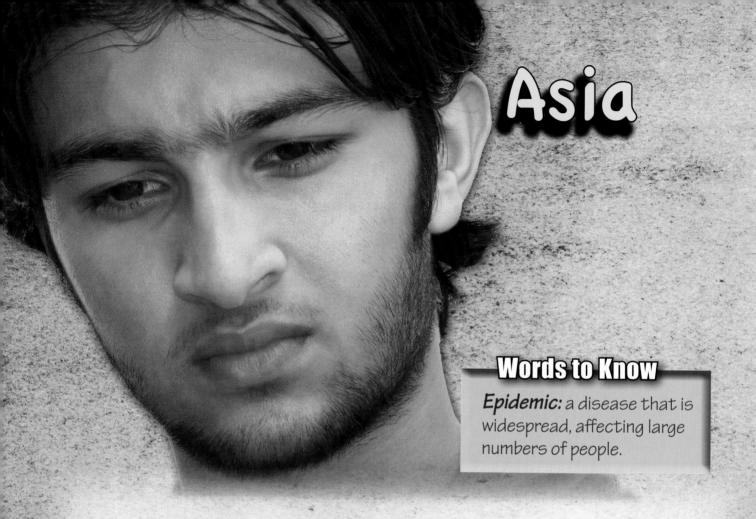

Asia

Asia has been hit hard by the AIDS epidemic. More AIDS deaths happen here than anywhere else in the world except Africa. Russia has almost no AIDS education program at all, but India is the Asian country with the most people who have HIV.

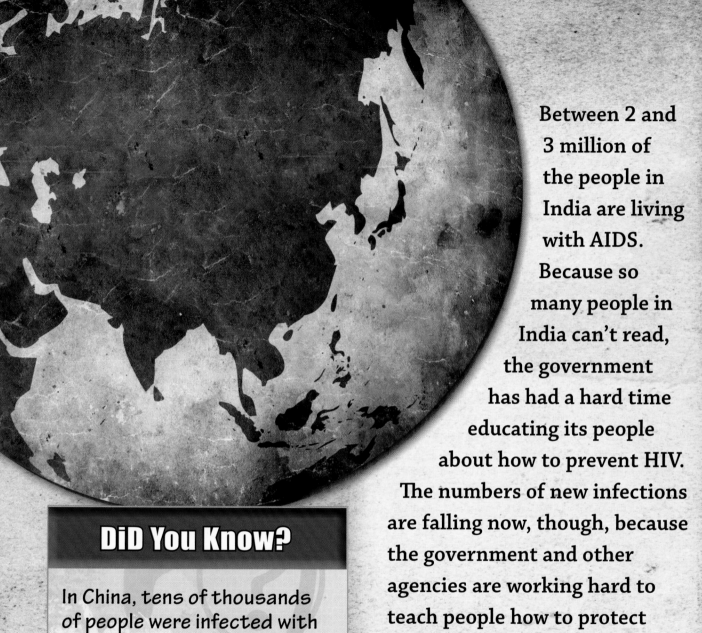

Between 2 and 3 million of the people in India are living with AIDS. Because so many people in India can't read, the government has had a hard time educating its people about how to prevent HIV. The numbers of new infections are falling now, though, because the government and other agencies are working hard to teach people how to protect themselves.

DiD You Know?

In China, tens of thousands of people were infected with HIV from blood transfusions that had been donated by people who had HIV.

Europe and . . . .

Western Europe is doing everything it can to educate people about how to keep themselves safe from the HIV virus. HIV medicines are available, and the death rate has fallen.

Eastern Europe, however, is not doing as well. There are many new countries in that region who are struggling to build their governments and economies. HIV puts an added strain on them that is hard for them to handle.

Australia recognized and responded to AIDS earlier and more quickly than many regions of the world. It has one of the most successful HIV prevention and health education programs in the world. Its HIV infection rates are fairly low as a result.

Australia

Words to Know

Economies: systems for handling money and the production of wealth.

South America

AIDS is a serious problem in South America, just as it is in the rest of the world. Brazil, the largest nation in South America, has launched a powerful campaign against HIV/AIDS.

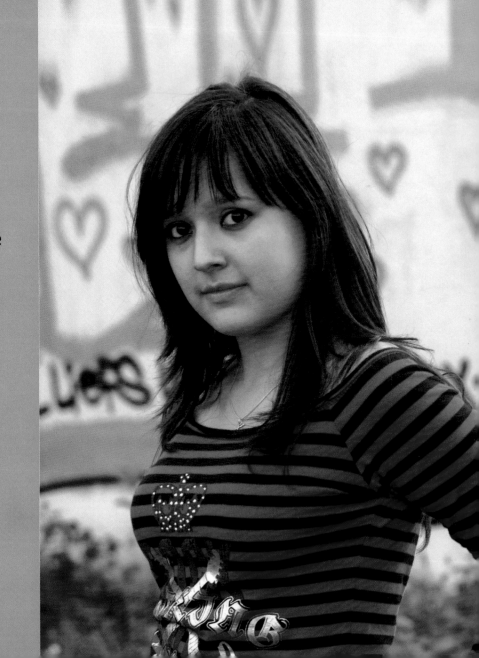

One of the things that Brazil does is hand out clean hypodermic needles for free. The government is also teaching its people other ways to protect themselves. HIV drugs are cheap in Brazil, so that everyone can afford to be treated.

Not everyone in the world approves of Brazil's approach to AIDS. Some people think it's not fair to the drug companies that make the drugs if Brazil sells the medicine so cheaply. Other people say that by handing out clean needles, the government is saying it's okay to do drugs.

What Is the World Doing to Fight AIDS?

All over the world, AIDS is affecting the lives of human beings, people not so different from you. And now people all over the world are joining the fight against AIDS.

Words to Know

Solidarity: agreement and support between people.

48

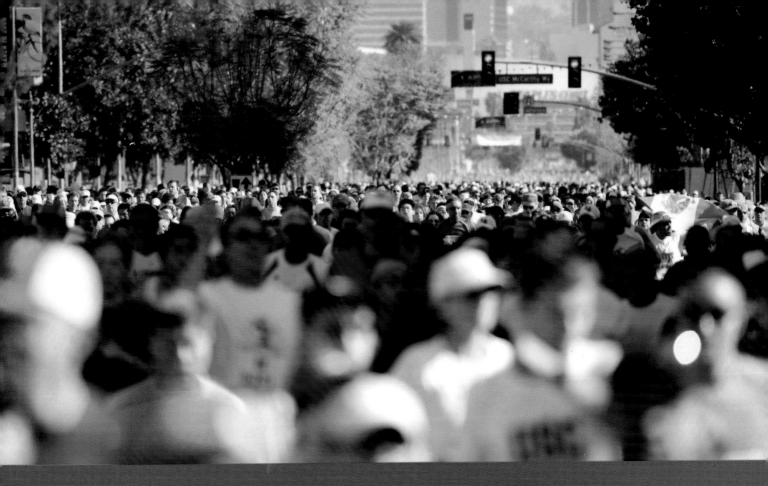

Most of these people have names you've probably never heard—
but many of them are famous people who use their position to bring
more attention to the cause they've taken on. From the ordinary
people who take part in AIDS marathons like the one shown here to
hip-hop artists and fashion models, movie stars to talk show hosts,
more and more people are getting involved. The red ribbon has
become the symbol that stands for people's solidarity with all those
who are living with HIV/AIDS.

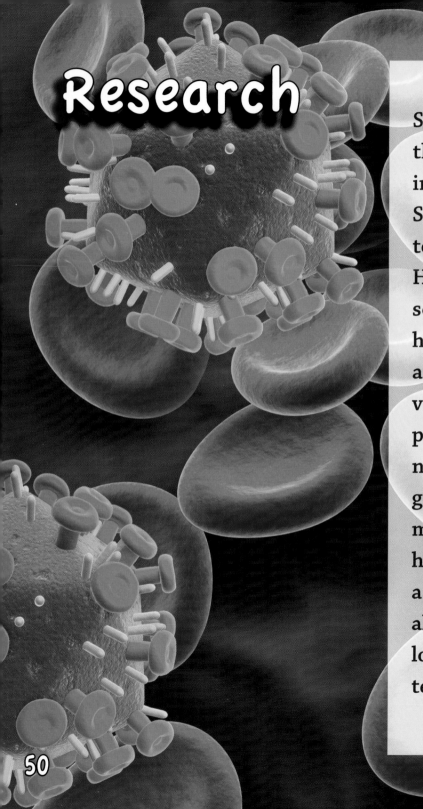

Research

Scientific research is one of the most powerful weapons in the battle against AIDS. Scientists are working hard to find new ways to treat HIV and slow its progress so people can live longer, healthier lives. Researchers are also trying to create a vaccine against HIV, so that people could get a shot and never have to worry about getting this disease. And most of all, scientists are hoping to someday find a way to cure HIV/AIDS altogether, so people will no longer have to die from this terrible disease.

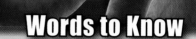

Vaccine: a substance that prevents a particular disease by helping your immune system fight off an enemy (such as a virus, a bacteria, or cancer).

Reseach takes lots of money. The scientists who work on this problem need to be paid. Their equipment and materials are expensive. And their job takes lots of time. There aren't any easy, quick answers!

Some organizations are helping to raise money for AIDS research. Many people believe governments should be spending more on research to finally find a cure.

The United Nations

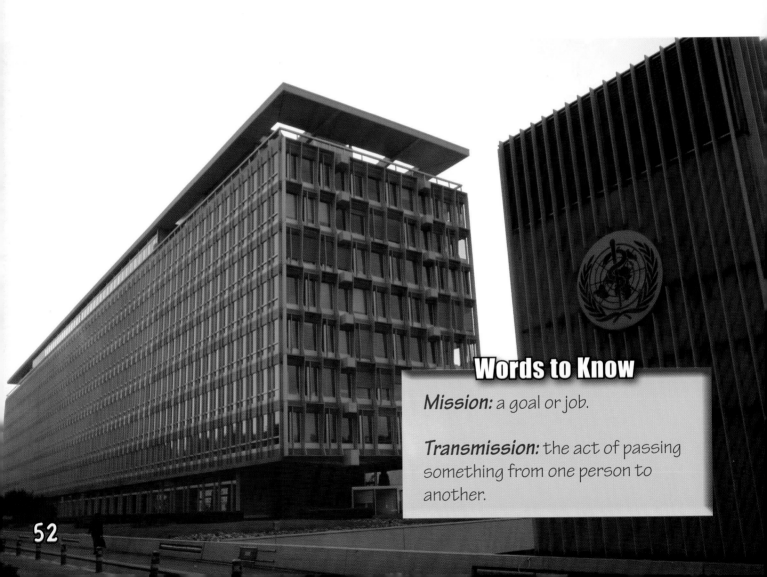

Words to Know

Mission: a goal or job.

Transmission: the act of passing something from one person to another.

In September 2000, 189 of the world's nations met for the United Nations' Millennium Summit. One of the goals they set themselves was to combat HIV/AIDS. The United Nations set up a special agency to do this job called UNAIDS. Its mission includes:

- preventing the transmission of HIV
- providing care and support to those already living with the virus
- working to make individuals and communities stronger, so they won't be as apt to get HIV
- helping countries cope with the costs of HIV/AIDS (both in terms of money and in human life)

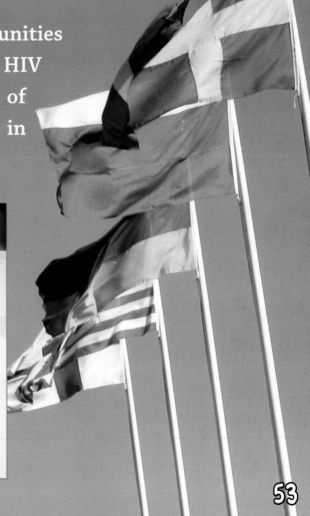

DiD You Know?

The World Health Organization (its headquarters in Geneva, Switzerland, is shown to the left) is the part of the United Nations that works especially with anything that has to do with health.

The United Nations began in 1945 as a group of countries that got together to work for the peace and well-being of the entire world.

(PRODUCT) RED

One of the stars who's leading the battle against AIDS is Bono from the rock group U2. In 1986, Bono went to Ethiopia, a country in Africa. There Bono was faced with thousands of sick and hungry people. As Bono talked to these people, he felt angry that they had to live in such terrible conditions. Today, he's still angry, and he uses his anger to make himself fight hard against AIDS. Bono is famous around the world not only because he's a rock star, but also because he's someone who speaks out on behalf of those who are living with HIV/AIDS.

Bono doesn't just talk. He uses his position to take action. One thing he did was to help start a line of products called (PRODUCT) RED. These include everything from laptops to iPods®, T-shirts to jeans. A part of the sales from each of these products goes to the Global Fund, an organization that fights AIDS. Bono explained, "Now you're buying jeans and T-shirts, and you're paying for 10 women in Africa to get medication for their children with HIV."

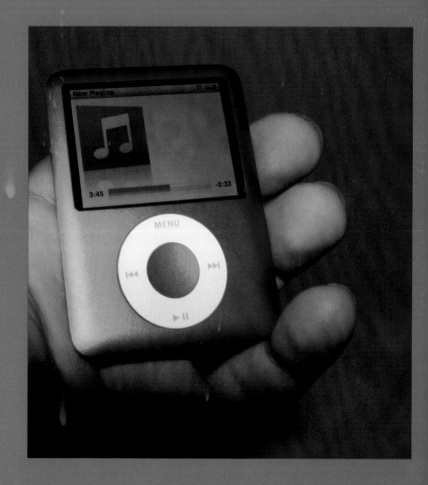

What Can You Do to Stay Safe?

The only way to be sure you won't catch HIV/AIDS is to protect yourself from other people's body fluids.

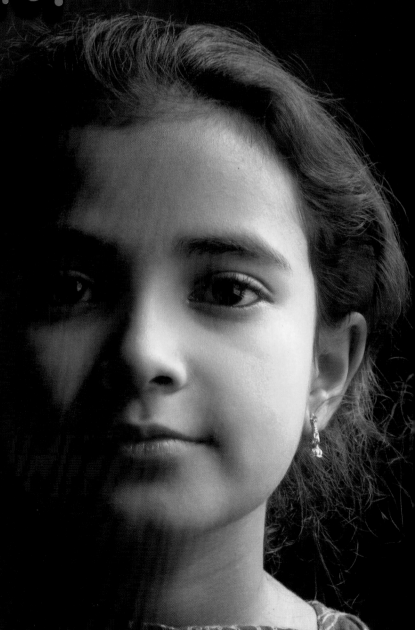

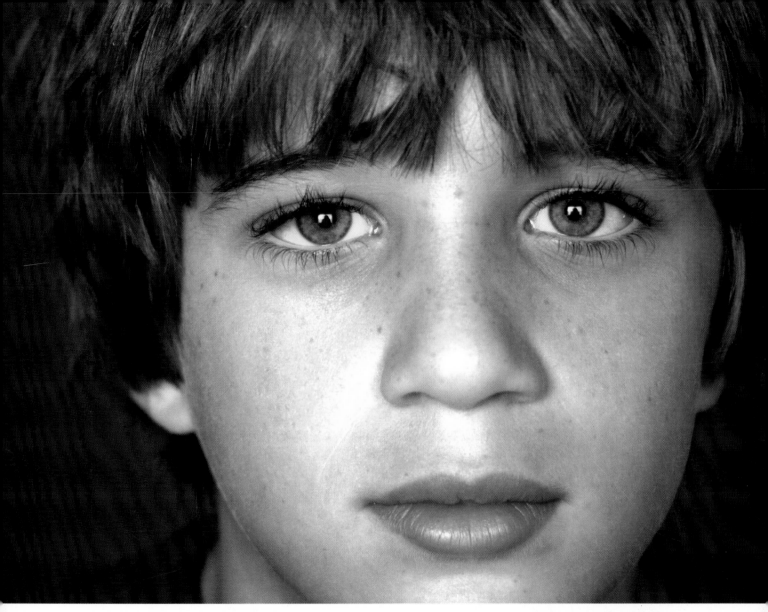

Sex is the way most people come into contact with body fluids, and condoms can help protect them. Also be careful not to touch another person's sores or blood. Pass the word. Tell your friends what they can do to stay safe. And join the people who are fighting HIV/AIDS. Do whatever you can!

57

Real Kids

Ryan White began 1984 as an ordinary thirteen-year-old. He had hemophilia, but it was being treated. He went to school and had friends, just like most kids his age. Then Ryan and his family found out he had caught HIV through the blood he had received to treat his hemophilia. The HIV had already advanced to AIDS. Doctors told Ryan and his family that he only had six months to live.

Ryan wanted to spend the last months of his life doing what he had been doing, going to school and being with friends. But the school didn't want him there. People were afraid Ryan's illness might "rub off" on the other students.

Ryan's battle to be allowed to attend school made news first in the United States and then around the world. Because of Ryan, people all over the world started thinking about AIDS.

On April 8, 1990, Ryan White lost his battle with AIDS. He was only nineteen when he died, but he had done a lot with his life. Because he fought hard to make people realize that AIDS is a problem we must all face, laws were passed to help people with HIV/AIDS, television shows were made, magazine articles were written, and education programs were started in schools. The world began to work together to fight this terrible disease—all because one young boy was brave enough to take a stand.

Find Out More

These books and Web sites will tell you more about HIV/AIDS, what you can do to protect yourself, and how you can help fight this disease.

The AIDS Handbook: Written for Middle School Kids by Middle School Kids
www.eastchester.k12.ny.us/schools/ms/AIDS/AIDS1.html

Let's Talk: Children, Families, and HIV
www.kidstalkaids.org/education/index.html

The Millennium Project
www.millenniumproject.org

NGOs International HIV/AIDS Alliance
www.aidsalliance.org/sw7119.asp

ONE
www.one.org

YouthAIDS (What You Can Do to Change the World)
www.youthaids.org

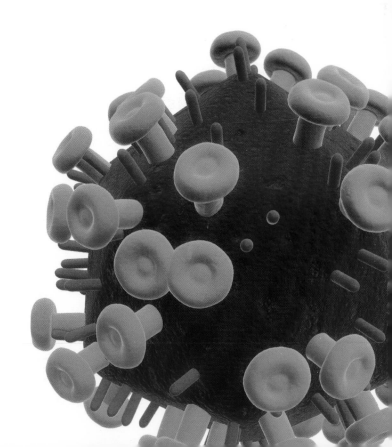

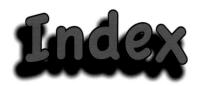

Index

Picture Credits

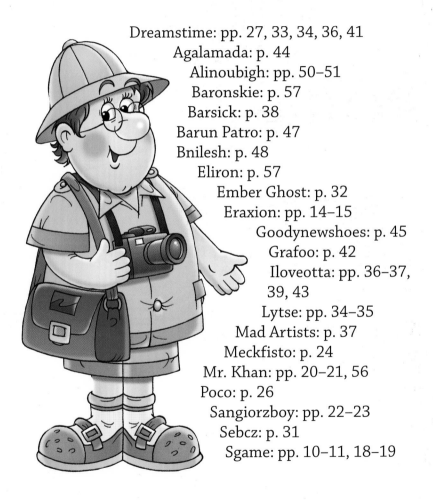

Dreamstime: pp. 27, 33, 34, 36, 41
Agalamada: p. 44
Alinoubigh: pp. 50–51
Baronskie: p. 57
Barsick: p. 38
Barun Patro: p. 47
Bnilesh: p. 48
Eliron: p. 57
Ember Ghost: p. 32
Eraxion: pp. 14–15
Goodynewshoes: p. 45
Grafoo: p. 42
Iloveotta: pp. 36–37, 39, 43
Lytse: pp. 34–35
Mad Artists: p. 37
Meckfisto: p. 24
Mr. Khan: pp. 20–21, 56
Poco: p. 26
Sangiorzboy: pp. 22–23
Sebcz: p. 31
Sgame: pp. 10–11, 18–19

Streetgraphics: p. 46
Volspale: p. 40, 45
Yanc: pp.34–35
Yurok: pp. 34–35
iStockphotos
Mickel, Felix: pp. 32–33
(Product) Red: pp. 54, 55
United Nations: p. 52

To the best knowledge of the publisher, all other images are in the public domain. If any image has been inadvertently uncredited, please notify Harding House Publishing Service, Vestal, New York 13850, so that rectification can be made for future printings.

About the Author

Rae Simons has written many books for young adults and children. She lives with her family in New York State in the U.S.

About the Consultant

Elise DeVore Berlan, MD, MPH, FAAP, is a faculty member of the Division of Adolescent Health at Nationwide Children's Hospital and an Assistant Professor of Clinical Pediatrics at The Ohio State University College of Medicine. She completed her Fellowship in Adolescent Medicine at Children's Hospital Boston and obtained a Master's Degree in Public Health at the Harvard School of Public Health. Dr. Berlan completed her residency in pediatrics at the Children's Hospital of Philadelphia, where she also served an additional year as Chief Resident. She received her medical degree from the University of Iowa College of Medicine.